First, the facts...

1 The menopause is your last menstrual period. It marks the end of your reproductive years and the start of a new phase of life.

2 Many women experience symptoms as they near the menopause – this time of life is known as the perimenopause or menopause transition.

3 The average age at which women start the menopause transition is 46 years. Periods usually stop by the age of 51.

4 The most common symptoms are heavy bleeding, hot flushes, night sweats, emotional instability, vaginal dryness and bladder problems. Symptoms can range from mild to debilitating.

5 Much can be done to help with symptoms during the menopause transition, including lifestyle changes, hormone replacement therapy (HRT) and treatments for individual symptoms.

6 For women under 60 years of age who are in good health, the benefits of HRT far outweigh any risks.

This book provides the information you need to have an informed discussion with your healthcare professional and to help you choose how you want to manage your menopause transition. Spaces have been provided to help you keep notes on your symptoms and concerns and record any questions you may have.

My main concerns

Make a note of anything you want to discuss with your doctor here…

T0018756

What is the menopause?

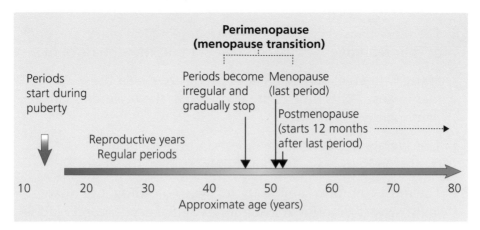

The menopause is specifically your last menstrual period. However, the word menopause is widely used to describe the time around this event when many women experience symptoms. This is more accurately known as the **perimenopause**. It can be thought of as the **menopause transition** (gradual change) from the reproductive years to the postmenopausal years, and this is the term most frequently used in this book.

During the menopause transition, the amount of oestrogen produced by the ovaries changes (see page 5). Instead of having a regular menstrual cycle, it becomes unpredictable. The changing levels of oestrogen cause symptoms, such as heavy bleeding, hot flushes, night sweats, emotional instability, vaginal dryness and bladder problems.

> **TERMINOLOGY TIP**
>
> **Perimenopausal** means the time around the menopause ('peri' means 'around'). This period of **menopause transition** is the gradual change as your periods stop through to 12 months after your last period.
>
> **Postmenopausal** means the time from 12 months after your last period ('post' means 'after').

When does the menopause happen?

- The average age for the start of the menopause transition is 46 years – much younger than most women expect.
- Perimenopausal symptoms that start before the age of 45 are referred to as early menopause.
- The menopause itself is reached when the ovaries stop producing oestrogen.
- The postmenopause starts 12 months after a woman's last period. Periods usually stop by the age of 51, so the average age for becoming postmenopausal in the UK is 52.

We can't predict when a woman will reach the menopause transition. It is not related to the age she started her periods. However, there may be an inherited aspect, so if your mother had an early natural menopause, you may too.

> Although we talk about 'averages' here, there is no 'normal' or 'average'. The age at which the menopause transition starts and finishes varies widely, as do the symptoms women experience, how mild or severe they are, and how long they last.

My notes

Make a note here of key dates (for example, when you think your symptoms started, when you get your periods, or the age at which your mother went through the menopause)...

What's happening with my hormones?

During your reproductive years

The menstrual cycle is a complex process, regulated by hormones.

When you are born, your ovaries contain lots of eggs (ova). From puberty, most of the time an egg matures each month and is released. This process is controlled by two hormones that are released by the pituitary gland – follicle-stimulating hormone (FSH) and luteinising hormone (LH). FSH and LH also stimulate the ovaries to produce the hormones oestrogen and progesterone.

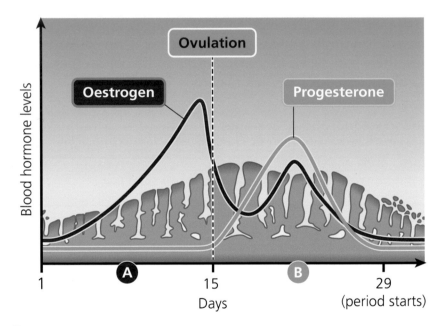

A In the first phase of the menstrual cycle, the ovaries release oestrogen, which causes the lining of the uterus (womb) to thicken.

B After ovulation (which is when the egg is released), rising levels of progesterone prepare the lining of the womb to receive a fertilised egg.

If the egg is not fertilised, levels of progesterone and oestrogen decrease and the lining of the womb is shed – this is your period.

The menopause transition

As you get older, your ovaries may not release an egg in every cycle. As a result, levels of both oestrogen and progesterone vary unpredictably.

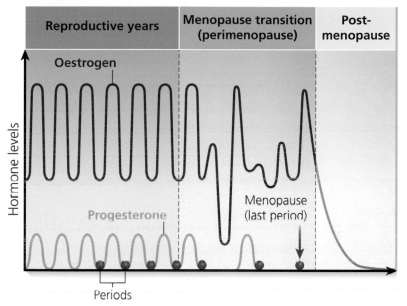

Reproductive years	Menopause transition (perimenopause)	Post-menopause

Oestrogen

Hormone levels

Progesterone

Menopause (last period)

Periods

These unpredictable hormone levels cause the symptoms of the menopause transition. During this time, the lining of the womb may become too thick and is shed in a disordered way, resulting in irregular, heavy periods (see page 13).

After the menopause

After the menopause, oestrogen levels are very low and women generally experience fewer symptoms – although some women continue to have symptoms such as hot flushes.

Most importantly, the falling level of oestrogen increases the risk of cardiovascular disease (CVD) and osteoporosis. Lack of oestrogen also affects the condition of the vaginal and bladder tissues.

These are important issues to consider, regardless of your symptoms during the menopause transition, because you could live for 30 years in the postmenopausal period. We talk about this on pages 26–7.

Other reasons for menopause

Some women will experience menopause for reasons other than natural ageing. These include premature ovarian insufficiency or a chronic health condition that causes early menopause, or removal of their ovaries to reduce their risk of certain cancers or to alleviate pain associated with endometriosis.

Surgical menopause

Women who have their ovaries removed as part of a subtotal or radical hysterectomy (removal of the womb and some associated tissues) can experience an abrupt onset of menopausal symptoms. Your healthcare professional should discuss ways to manage these symptoms before you have surgery and put in place an individualised treatment plan, guided by your medical history.

Most women can start HRT immediately after surgery. This is best delivered through the skin to prevent any increase in the risk of blood clots in the legs or lungs. Oestrogen-only HRT is most common, but you may also need a progestogen for the first 12 months or longer if you have endometriosis or if your cervix was not removed as part of your surgery.

Ovaries that are not removed during a hysterectomy often fail early. You can consider using HRT as soon as you experience symptoms.

If you are over 45 years of age when your ovaries stop producing hormones reliably, you will not need a blood test and you can start HRT without delay after consulting your healthcare professional. Again, if you have endometriosis or you still have your cervix, you may also need a progestogen.

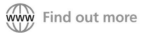 **Find out more**

www.womens-health-concern.org/help-and-advice/factsheets/induced
-menopause-in-women-with-endometriosis

www.menopausedoctor.co.uk/menopause/surgical-menopause-and-
menopause-in-women-with-endometriosis-video

Endometriosis

Endometriosis arises when tissue that is similar to the tissue that lines the womb (endometrium) grows in other places in the body. Common sites include:

- the ovaries, resulting in 'chocolate' cysts
- the Fallopian tubes, where it can cause fertility problems
- the lining of the abdominal cavity (this is called the peritoneum; it covers, supports and protects the organs inside the abdomen and pelvis)
- the muscle of the womb (in this location the condition is known as adenomyosis).

Less common sites include the belly button (which will bleed monthly), nose (monthly nose bleeds), lungs (monthly coughing of blood) and caesarean section scars (monthly pain).

Laparoscopy (keyhole surgery) is used to diagnose endometriosis. A small telescope is inserted into the abdomen via small incisions to look inside the body. The condition can be treated medically (often with hormones) or the deposits of endometriosis can be removed and/or scar tissue (adhesions) released during laparoscopy.

It is important that your healthcare professional considers your history of endometriosis when discussing your menopause management. If you have had surgical treatment, there may still be deposits of tissue in your body and you will need a progestogen to reduce the risk of hyperplasia (excess thickening of the tissue, which is a risk factor for cancer).

You may be eligible for a Mirena IUS (intrauterine system) if you have an intact uterus (that is, you have not had a hysterectomy). The progestogen released by the IUS will stop the endometrial tissue from thickening, no matter where in the body it is growing.

There are no clear guidelines on how long you will need a progestogen. Many clinicians recommend long-term use to reduce risk.

Premature ovarian insufficiency

Premature ovarian insufficiency (sometimes referred to as POI) occurs when the ovaries fail early (or are surgically removed) in women under the age of 40. There is usually no recognisable cause and it is particularly devastating in younger women who have not yet had children.

Women with POI are at increased risk of osteoporosis and CVD.

Following an individualised risk assessment, you may be offered either combined hormonal contraception – pill, patch or vaginal ring – or HRT.

Fertility treatment using a donor egg is an option for women who wish to become pregnant.

Chronic diseases

The menopause sometimes starts early in women with long-term (chronic) diseases, such as kidney failure, underactive thyroid, rheumatoid arthritis, epilepsy and migraine. Blood tests are recommended in women below the age of 40 (FSH should be checked on two separate occasions, 2–6 weeks apart). HRT is not completely off limits to women with underlying health issues, but it is best delivered through the skin as a patch, gel or spray rather than taken orally.

Women with asthma may notice a change in symptom control around the menopause transition. HRT can also affect symptom control: sometimes it helps, but sometimes control deteriorates. It is important that you discuss any problems with your healthcare professional.

Find out more

www.daisynetwork.org **(POI)**

www.asthma.org.uk/advice/manage-your-asthma/women/#painrelief **(HRT and asthma)**

How will the menopause transition affect me?

The menopause transition affects different women in different ways. There are lots of possible symptoms – you may not have any of them or you may have some or all of them, some or all of the time. Use the table on page 10 to keep a track of your symptoms. The most common symptoms are listed at the top of the table.

These are largely considered to be short-term symptoms – although some women continue to experience some of these symptoms for many years.

Note that poor sleep in a previously good sleeper is a common but subtle early sign of the menopause transition.

We discuss how to manage these symptoms on pages 13–23.

A national survey conducted on behalf of the British Menopause Society (BMS) found that one-half of women go through the menopause without consulting a healthcare professional – even though 42% said that symptoms were worse than expected. Half the women said that the menopause had affected their home life, and one-third said it had affected their work life.

My questions

Is there anything you don't understand about the menopause transition? Write your questions here, so that you can ask your doctor...

My menopausal symptoms

Use this table to keep track of your symptoms over 2–3 weeks. Make a note of the severity of your symptoms – mild: 1, moderate: 2, severe: 3 – and how long the symptoms last.

Week beginning:			
Heavy bleeding			
Hot flushes			
Night sweats			
Vaginal dryness			
Emotional instability (e.g. irritation, tearfulness)			
Bladder problems*			
Poor sleep			
Forgetfulness			
Poor concentration			
Difficulty coping			
Lack of drive			
Anxiety			
Depression			
Changes to the hair			
Changes to the skin			
Loss of interest in sex (low libido)			
Joint pains			
Muscle pains			
Headaches			
Palpitations (racing heart)			
Other...			

*Urgent need to pass urine, incontinence, overactive bladder.

Q: How do I know if I have started the menopause transition?

If you are aged 40–50, have any of the symptoms on page 10 and your periods are irregular, you are likely to be in the menopause transition.

Q: Do I need a blood test?

Most women do not need a blood test. However, if you are younger than 40 and have perimenopausal symptoms, your doctor will recommend that you have two blood tests 6 weeks apart to measure the levels of FSH. High levels of FSH may indicate premature ovarian insufficiency, which should be treated with HRT.

Q: I've had a hysterectomy. How will the menopause affect me?

Perimenopausal symptoms are caused by changes in the hormones released from the ovaries (see page 5). If you have had a hysterectomy (removal of the womb) but still have your ovaries, you may get perimenopausal symptoms (except heavy bleeding). However, the symptoms may start earlier than in women who still have a womb.

Women who start taking HRT after a hysterectomy and possibly after an oophorectomy (removal of the ovaries) can continue taking it to age 60 (and beyond if needed) to control menopausal symptoms.

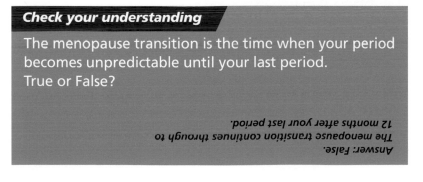

Check your understanding

The menopause transition is the time when your period becomes unpredictable until your last period.
True or False?

Answer: False.
The menopause transition continues through to 12 months after your last period.

Q: **I take the combined contraceptive pill. How will the menopause affect me?**

Every woman will reach the menopause. However, if you are taking a combined hormonal contraceptive, the perimenopausal symptoms may be masked and you may not know exactly when you reach the menopause.

For women under 50, combined hormonal contraception (pills, patches and vaginal rings) can help control perimenopausal symptoms (including heavy periods).

You can take combined oral contraception ('the pill') until age 50. You will then need to change to a progestogen-only contraceptive method until age 55.

The Mirena IUS can be combined with oestrogen-only HRT to help with perimenopausal symptoms in addition to providing contraception.

Q: **I don't have periods because I have a progestogen-based IUS. How will the menopause affect me?**

Perimenopausal symptoms are caused by changes in the levels of hormones released from the ovaries, so although you have an IUS you may still have perimenopausal symptoms (except heavy bleeding).

The Mirena IUS can be used as part of HRT to protect the lining of the womb (it provides the progestogen component). It is usually replaced every 5 years.

TERMINOLOGY TIP

Progesterone is a naturally occurring hormone (see pages 4–5).

Progestogens (sometimes called progestins) are synthetic forms of progesterone.

Managing the common symptoms

Heavy bleeding

Irregular or heavy bleeding is often an early symptom of the menopause transition (see page 5). You may have less of a gap between heavier periods, or you may go for several months without a period.

Bleeding is unacceptable if it is heavy for you, regardless of the amount of blood you lose or how much sanitary protection you require.

Practical tips

❏ Keep a track of your periods for discussion with your doctor. Make a note of: when they start, how long they last, how heavy they are, any spotting in between periods, and any abnormal bleeding, pain, discomfort or other symptoms.

❏ Wear panty liners or protective underwear if the timing of your periods is unpredictable.

❏ Use high-absorbency tampons or pads during your period and change them every 2–4 hours.

❏ Keep using contraception if you are under the age of 55. You can get pregnant during the menopause transition.

Further steps if needed

❏ Talk to your doctor if you are concerned about heavy bleeding to rule out other causes, such as fibroids.

❏ Talk to your doctor if you are feeling tired or look paler than usual. You may have anaemia. Your doctor can do a blood test and may give you iron tablets.

❏ Non-steroidal anti-inflammatory drugs, such as ibuprofen, can help with menstrual cramps and may reduce your flow by up to 30%.

❏ An IUS that contains 52 mg of the progestogen levonorgestrel reduces bleeding in most women without changing the menstrual cycle. Only the Mirena IUS is licensed for use as part of HRT.

Hot flushes

Hot flushes are a sudden feeling of intense heat that spreads throughout the body. They may last seconds or minutes, and may be accompanied by reddening of the skin, sweating and sometimes palpitations (rapid heart rate). Hot flushes can lead to embarrassment and anxiety.

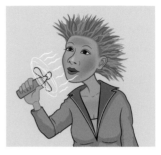

Hot flushes are one of the most common and well-known symptoms of the menopause transition. In the BMS survey (see page 9), 79% of women aged 45–65 experienced hot flushes.

In general, women get hot flushes for an average of 5 years, although it can be a lot longer than this. Some women experience very few, whereas others may get several hot flushes a day.

Practical tips

❏ Wear several thin layers of clothing, and choose clothes that you can remove quickly and easily.

❏ Carry a fan with you, or try neck-cooling scarves/bandanas.

❏ Cool your face with cold water if you feel a hot flush coming on.

❏ Avoid triggers such as spicy food, alcohol and caffeine.

❏ Check whether any medicine you are taking increases the risk of hot flushes; talk to your doctor if you think this is an issue.

❏ Use relaxation and breathing techniques to avoid stress and anxiety, as they can make hot flushes worse.

Further steps if needed

☐ HRT is the recommended treatment for hot flushes and is highly effective (see pages 28–41).

☐ Femal (bee pollen) has been shown to reduce hot flushes.

☐ Your doctor may prescribe medications called SSRIs or SNRIs (selective serotonin- or norepinephrine-reuptake inhibitors). These medications are used to treat depression but can also reduce perimenopausal symptoms. An SSRI may be helpful if HRT is not an option.

☐ Pregabalin, gabapentin and clonidine may also help to reduce hot flushes. All these medications have other uses.

Night sweats

Night sweats are hot flushes that happen during the night. They can disturb your sleep pattern (and your partner's), resulting in tiredness. Some women may have difficulty coping because of lack of sleep.

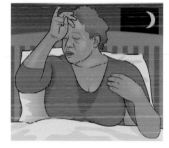

In the BMS survey (see page 9), 70% of women reported having night sweats.

Practical tips

☐ Wear fewer and/or looser clothes at night.

☐ Have two single duvets on your bed, so that you and your partner can each choose the level of warmth that works for you.

☐ Try a cooling pillow.

☐ Look out for triggers, such as spicy food, alcohol and caffeine.

- [ ] Check whether any of your medications are associated with night sweats; talk to your doctor if you think this is an issue.
- [ ] Try not to worry about how much sleep you are getting.

Further steps if needed
- [ ] HRT is highly effective in controlling night sweats and improving sleep patterns (see pages 28–41).

Managing my symptoms

Make a note here if you have been experiencing hot flushes or night sweats. Include when the symptoms occur, possible triggers and any practical tips you have tried.

Vaginal dryness

Instead of being stretchy and well lubricated, the tissues of the vagina become dry and are more easily damaged. The terminology for this may be confusing but the author's preferred term is 'urogenital atrophy'.

Vaginal dryness is a very common symptom of the menopause transition, but women are often embarrassed to talk about it.

Urogenital atrophy may cause discomfort or pain during sex. It can also make a smear test difficult or painful.

In the BMS survey (see page 9), 35% of women said they had experienced vaginal dryness, with 18% of those who had this symptom saying it was unexpected.

Practical tips
☐ Use lubricants during sex.

☐ Try vaginal moisturisers, available from pharmacies.

Further steps if needed
☐ Your doctor can prescribe vaginal moisturisers, which can be used twice weekly to reduce vaginal dryness.

☐ Your doctor can also prescribe treatments that deliver low doses of oestrogen directly to the vagina. These are available as pessaries, creams or a vaginal ring.

☐ Another treatment option is prasterone, a pessary inserted into the vagina on a daily basis. It releases a precursor hormone (dehydroepiandrosterone or DHEA), which is converted in the lining of the vagina to oestrogen and testosterone with virtually no absorption into the bloodstream. Both oestrogen and testosterone are important for tissue quality.

☐ In general, urogenital atrophy is best managed with treatments that are delivered directly to the vagina.

❏ If these treatments do not work, your doctor may prescribe a drug called ospemifene. It is taken by mouth and improves tissue quality. It should be used alone, not added to HRT.

❏ It is important to keep using whatever your doctor has prescribed for vaginal dryness for several months. Some products can be used for life.

❏ If you are due for a smear test, use of these treatments for 3–6 months beforehand will help make the procedure easier. (It is important that you continue to have regular smear tests.)

Bladder problems

During the menopause transition you may experience a sudden or constant need to pass urine (urge incontinence), leakages during exercise or when laughing or coughing (stress incontinence), or both of these (mixed incontinence). You may also find that it is painful to pass urine.

A lack of oestrogen causes the tissues in your vagina and urethra (the tube that carries urine out of the body) to lose their elasticity. The pelvic floor may also weaken.

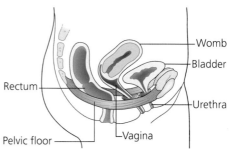

- Getting older also has various debilitating effects on the pelvic organs and tissues.

- When you are standing, most of your bodyweight bears down on the pelvic floor, so being overweight makes this worse.

- Pregnancy and childbirth put pressure on the pelvic floor, especially if a baby was large, labour was prolonged or instruments were used to help the delivery.

- Coughing and constipation can also stress the pelvic floor.

- Some women have poor-quality tissue for genetic reasons.

- The bladder tissues are also affected by oestrogen, so bladder problems can occur during and after the menopause transition.

- Overactive bladder can increase the need to pass urine, including during the night, which disrupts sleep.

> **TERMINOLOGY TIP**
>
> The **pelvic floor** is a 'sling' of muscle and fibrous tissue that supports your bladder and other organs.

Practical tips

☐ Pelvic floor exercises (also called Kegel exercises) strengthen the pelvic floor and can therefore help with bladder control. These exercises can also increase sexual pleasure.

> It is never too soon or too late to start these exercises!

- You can identify the muscles of your pelvic floor by squeezing around your back passage as though trying to stop wind and at the same time squeezing at the front as if trying to stop passing urine. The front and back contract at the same time.

- Exercising these muscles can help to prevent bladder problems and reduce problems that already exist.

- Many resources and apps are available to help you learn how to do these exercises and to remind you to do them (forever). For example, the NHS Apps Library recommends the inexpensive 'Squeezy' app (www.squeezyapp.com)

- Ask your doctor to refer you to a specialist physiotherapist if you feel that you need more help.

☐ Other forms of exercise can strengthen the pelvic floor, particularly yoga and Pilates.

☐ Have your last drink at least 1 hour before going to bed.

☐ Try to reduce your intake of caffeine and alcohol, as these can worsen symptoms.

☐ Try to avoid spicy foods as these may also irritate the bladder.

Further steps if needed

❑ Your doctor can prescribe various treatments to improve urogenital tissue quality (see pages 17–18) in addition to a medication for overactive bladder.

❑ Additional oral medication may be required for women with overactive bladder or mixed incontinence.

Managing my symptoms

Make a note here if you have been experiencing vaginal dryness or bladder problems. Write down any questions you want to ask your doctor.

Effects on your mood and mind

You may experience changing emotions (emotional lability) at this time of life for many reasons, but the changes in hormones during the menopause transition may make this worse.

Common emotional issues include irritability, such as snapping for no apparent reason, low mood, anxiety, difficulty coping, lack of motivation, tearfulness and worsening phobias.

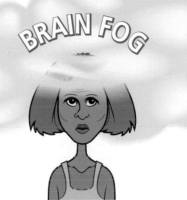

Lack of sleep – because of anxiety or night sweats – can make these symptoms worse.

Some women also report becoming more forgetful, poor concentration and 'brain fog'.

Women who are prone to mood changes are more likely to experience emotional lability during the menopause transition. Premenstrual symptoms may be worse during the menopause transition.

Practical tips

❑ Look after your general health and wellbeing, as described on page 25. This will help improve your mood.

❑ Try to exercise regularly; it is a particularly good way to improve your mood, as is being outdoors.

❑ Try relaxation techniques, breathing exercises and/or mindfulness. These can all help.

❏ Take time to look after yourself, away from the stresses of life and the demands of others.

❏ Tell your partner and family why you are feeling irritable. They are likely to be more supportive if they understand what you are going through.

❏ If these (or other symptoms) are affecting your work, talk to your human resources team (see page 43–4).

❏ Get support by talking to your friends and other women (see page 45).

Further steps if needed
If mood changes are affecting your quality of life, contact your doctor for help. There are a variety of treatments, including HRT and antidepressants (SSRIs and SNRIs, see page 15), that you can discuss.

Managing my symptoms

Make a note here if you have noticed any changes in your mood, concentration or memory. Write down any questions you want to ask your doctor.

Sex and the menopause

For some women the menopause represents freedom from periods and the worry of becoming pregnant. However, for others the hormone changes during the menopause transition can affect libido (interest in sex) and cause problems such as vaginal dryness (urogenital atrophy) and soreness, which can make sex difficult or painful. This may in turn reduce sexual desire and arousal, and reduce pleasure and orgasm.

The changes associated with urogenital atrophy may affect sexual intimacy and the ability to have a physical loving relationship. Women also report feeling less healthy and attractive. This can lead to avoidance of sex and intimacy – an important part of a relationship for many people.

Urogenital atrophy is also a common cause of bleeding after sex (postcoital bleeding).

 Warning: If you experience any bleeding after the menopause, see your doctor.

Practical tips
- ❏ Use lubricants to help during sex, and vaginal moisturisers to ease discomfort.
- ❏ Explore other types of stimulation and intimacy with your partner. Sex doesn't have to include penetration to be enjoyable.
- ❏ Find alternative ways to show affection and share intimacy with your partner. Even if you don't feel like having sex, affection and comfort are important and can help you feel better.

Further steps if needed
- ❏ Your doctor can prescribe various treatments to help with urogenital atrophy (see pages 17–18).

Do I need contraception during the menopause transition?

Yes! You can still get pregnant even if your periods are irregular, so you need to use contraception **until the age of 55**.

Once you reach 50, you should switch from a combined hormonal contraceptive to a progestogen-only method such as the 'mini-pill' or an IUS. This is because the combined pill contains a different type of oestrogen from HRT and is associated with more risks for women over the age of 50.

Managing my symptoms

Make a note here of any sexual problems you are experiencing, and practical tips you have tried...

Lifestyle changes to help manage symptoms

Many women find that changes to their daily lifestyle are helpful in reducing symptoms during the menopause transition. Begin with small changes, as these will be more manageable. You are also more likely to notice what helps, and to keep them up.

Consider getting more active and watching what you eat and drink.

- Physical activity will help with symptoms during the menopause transition and your general health and wellbeing. Weight-bearing activities (such as running and walking) are important to protect your bones. Activities such as yoga and Pilates are good for general strength and flexibility and improve the pelvic floor (see page 19), helping with continence.

- Plenty of advice is available about what to eat to maintain good health, and how much to eat. The key is to eat a wide variety of foods.

- Alcohol and caffeine can trigger hot flushes and may affect your sleep quality. Alcohol contains a lot of calories while caffeine is a diuretic, which means it increases the amount of urine you produce and therefore the number of times you need to pass urine. Coffee, tea and hot chocolate all contain caffeine.

---

www **Find out more**

- **The NHS site** www.nhs.uk/live-well/eat-well is a good starting point for finding out more about a healthy, balanced and sustainable diet

- The Change for Life website www.nhs.uk/change4life has lots of ideas for small lifestyle changes. Although it is intended for children, the advice and tips apply equally well to adults!

- www.menopausematters.co.uk/diet.php offers general information about diet, exercise and lifestyle during the menopause

- You can learn more about nutrition and exercise for bone health on the Royal Osteoporosis Society website www.theros.org.uk

Long-term consequences of the menopause

So far, we've talked about symptoms that may occur during the menopause transition (pages 13–22). However, it is also important to understand the long-term consequences of the menopause.

Oestrogen protects the cardiovascular system, bones, brain, and vaginal and bladder tissues. This protection is lost after the menopause, increasing the risk of CVD (heart attack and stroke), osteoporosis, cognitive decline, and vaginal and bladder problems.

While the menopause is inevitable, these long-term consequences are not. There are many ways to reduce the risk through lifestyle changes (page 25) and HRT (pages 28–41).

Cardiovascular disease

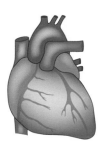

- Oestrogen protects the cardiovascular system (heart and blood vessels) during your reproductive years.
- This benefit is gradually lost after the menopause, which increases the risk of CVD, including heart attack and stroke.

  CVD is the leading cause of death in women over 50.

Osteoporosis

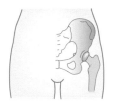

- Oestrogen protects the bones during your reproductive years.
- After the menopause, women lose about 1% of their bone density each year. This puts them at risk of fractures.
- Fractures related to osteoporosis are the most common cause of poor health in postmenopausal women.

Vaginal dryness

- Many women experience vaginal dryness during the menopause transition and postmenopausal years: instead of being stretchy and well lubricated, the tissues become dry and are more easily damaged.
- Vaginal dryness may cause discomfort or pain during sex and may make smear tests painful.

Bladder problems

- The bladder and other tissues in the urinary system are also affected by oestrogen levels. The changes in the vagina and urinary system are sometimes called urogenital atrophy.
- Many women experience bladder problems during the menopause transition and postmenopausal years. Problems include needing to pass urine more often (which may disturb sleep) and incontinence.

Cognitive decline

- Many women have problems with short-term memory and 'brain fog' during the menopause transition, but this usually improves after the menopause.
- The lack of oestrogen after the menopause may increase the risk of cognitive decline (decrease in memory and thinking skills) and possibly dementia.

My questions

Make a note here of any questions you have about the longer-term consequences of the menopause to ask your doctor...

Hormone replacement therapy

HRT replaces the oestrogen that you lose during the menopause transition, either alone or in combination with a progestogen. It helps to alleviate menopausal symptoms and also reduces the long-term consequences of the menopause (see pages 26–7).

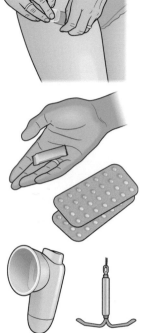

HRT is recommended as the best treatment for menopausal symptoms – based on all the available evidence.

There are many products and delivery options for HRT, including tablets, patches, gels, a spray and implants. This allows your HRT to be tailored to your needs. A patch, gel, spray or implant may be more suitable than tablets for some women, including those at risk of blood clots (see page 35). You may need to try more than one type of HRT to find the one that suits you.

HRT helps many women through their menopause transition, but it is not suitable for everyone.

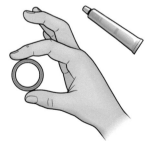

Some women are concerned about the apparent risks of HRT reported in the media. The benefits and risks of HRT are explained on pages 28–41 to help you decide whether you want to try HRT, and to help discussions with your doctor.

Check your understanding

HRT always contains oestrogen only. True or False?

Answer: False.
HRT can contain oestrogen alone or oestrogen and a progestogen.

Combined oestrogen and progestogen HRT

Women who have a womb and are still having periods (even if they are irregular) need HRT that contains a progestogen. This balances the effects of variable levels of oestrogen (as occurs during the menopause transition), as unopposed oestrogen can cause the lining of the womb to become too thick.

Many women start on a sequential preparation, which includes a progestogen for 12–14 days of each 28-day cycle, so that there is a monthly withdrawal bleed (as with the contraceptive pill). Sequential HRT can be delivered as tablets or through the skin (transdermally).

Preparations with less progestogen can be used, but bleeding may be heavy (although infrequent).

Women then move on to a **continuous combined oestrogen/ progestogen** product at about age 54. A progestogen is taken every day, so there is no monthly bleed. This 'bleed-free' HRT provides the best protection for the lining of the uterus in the long term. (It isn't used earlier in the menopause transition because it can cause irregular bleeding.) Continuous combined HRT is also delivered as tablets or through the skin.

Oestrogen-only HRT

This is suitable for women who:
- have had a total hysterectomy (removal of the womb and cervix)
- have had a Mirena IUS fitted within the last 5 years – Mirena contains the progestogen levonorgestrel which is released into the cavity of the womb, protecting the lining.

Phytoestrogens and other alternative therapies

Phytoestrogens are plant proteins that are similar to oestrogen, and they may help with symptoms during the menopause transition. They include soy products and isoflavones (red clover).

Evidence for the benefits of phytoestrogens in the menopause is mixed.

Red clover is more potent and better researched than soy, and some small studies have shown that it improves some symptoms in some women.

Red clover capsules are best taken at the time of day when symptoms are most troubling. They should not be taken by women with a risk or history of venous thromboembolism (see page 35) or hormone-sensitive cancers.

The use of black cohosh during the menopause is more controversial. It is approved for use in Germany as a non-prescription drug, but its effectiveness has not been proven. There are some concerns about its effects on the liver.

> When considering any form of **alternative therapy**, it is important to think about both the risks and the benefits, as you would for a medicine prescribed by a doctor. If you don't know whether something is likely to be beneficial, you may not want to expose yourself to even a low level of potential risk.

Testosterone

Testosterone is usually thought of as a male hormone; however, women also produce testosterone, but at much lower levels. Testosterone affects energy levels, sex drive (libido), muscles and joints. A woman's testosterone level decreases significantly as she gets older.

Testosterone can be used during the menopause transition to improve libido (interest in sex). A small amount of a testosterone gel (one-tenth of the dose used for men) is applied to the skin. It is best applied to areas of skin where there is no hair, such as the inner forearm. (Testosterone can cause hair growth if applied to areas of skin with hair follicles.)

There are currently no licensed products containing testosterone available on the NHS. Some GPs are reluctant to prescribe testosterone out of licence.

Weighing up the benefits and risks of HRT

When considering HRT, it is important to think about the benefits in terms of helping with symptoms during the menopause transition and the long-term benefits.

HRT protects against osteoporosis and CVD (depending on individual circumstances), and protects the vaginal and bladder tissues.

If you are under 60 and in good health, the benefits of HRT far outweigh the risks. However, the risks may be higher if you are overweight, smoke or have a family history of certain conditions. These risks need to be taken into account when considering which HRT is best for you.

Benefits	Risks
Short term • Controls symptoms during the menopause transition within days or weeks/improves mood **Long term** • Keeps bones healthy, reducing the risk of osteoporosis and fractures (broken bones) • Reduces the risk of CVD (as long as HRT is started within 5–6 years of the menopause transition and there are no other risk factors) • May protect against memory loss and possibly Alzheimer's disease • Reduces the risk of bowel cancer	• Oral HRT increases the risk of deep vein thrombosis (DVT) • Increases the risk of CVD in women who start HRT after age 60 and in those who already have risk factors, such as smoking, being overweight, or having high blood pressure or high cholesterol • Small increase in breast-cancer risk after age 60 (see pages 37–9) • Slight increase in the risk of gallbladder disease Note: some of these risks (for example, DVT) are not increased when oestrogen is administered by patch, gel or spray rather than as tablets.

The long-term benefits of HRT

Osteoporosis

Oestrogen is important for bone
health. Bone density decreases after
the menopause, increasing the risk of
osteoporosis (thinning of the bones).
This in turn increases the risk of fractures
(breaks), particularly of the hip, wrist
and vertebrae (the bones that make up
the spine). Osteoporosis affecting the
vertebrae can cause loss of height and
back pain.

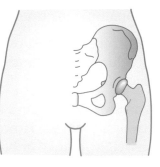

HRT reduces bone loss and the risk of fractures. A long-term US
study of 81 000 postmenopausal women showed that the risk of
hip fracture increased by 55% when women stopped taking HRT.

Women under 60 who have risk factors for osteoporosis (for
example, fracture or loss of height) or a family history of the
condition should consider HRT to reduce the risk of osteoporosis
and fractures.

TERMINOLOGY TIP

Osteoporosis means thinning of the bones. It particularly affects
the wrists, hip and spine.

- Regular weight-bearing exercise is important to keep your bones strong –
  walking, running or any other form of 'impact' exercise.

- It is also important that you have enough calcium and vitamin D in your
  diet, and exposure to sunlight, as these are also important for bone health.

Cardiovascular disease

CVD – which includes stroke and heart attack – is the leading cause of death in women over 50. Heart attack is the most common cause of death in postmenopausal women.

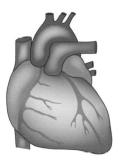

Lack of oestrogen after the menopause is one of several factors that increase the risk of CVD. Others include smoking, obesity, high blood pressure, diabetes and high cholesterol.

Oestrogen (either natural oestrogen before the menopause or the oestrogen in HRT) improves blood lipids (fats): it increases high-density ('good') cholesterol and decreases low-density ('bad') cholesterol. This protects against the development of atherosclerosis (a fatty layer in the blood vessels), which is the main cause of CVD.

Starting HRT within 5–6 years of the menopause protects against CVD: it reduces the risk of CVD by 40% and decreases the death rate from CVD. HRT also decreases the risk of stroke if started during the menopause transition.

As long as you start HRT early, you do not need to come off it at age 60, but it may increase the risk of CVD if started after age 60.

The beneficial effects appear to be greater in women who take oestrogen only.

Check your understanding

When do you need to start HRT for it to provide protection against CVD?

a) At the start of the menopause transition

b) During the menopause transition

c) After age 60

Answer: a) or b). HRT should be started within 5–6 years of the start of the menopause transition. Starting HRT after age 60 may increase the risk of CVD.

Arthritis

Oestrogen helps to maintain the cartilage that lines the bones in joints and the discs between the vertebrae in the spine.

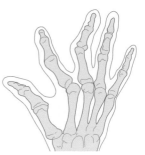

Cartilage can become thinner after the menopause, increasing the risk of arthritis and causing backache and other joint pain.

The oestrogen in HRT protects the cartilage, decreasing the risk and severity of arthritis. Progestogens seem to neutralise some of this benefit, but the Mirena IUS can be used to reduce the amount of progestogen in the bloodstream.

Memory and brain function

Long-term use of HRT within the first 5 years of the menopause has been shown to improve memory and reduce the incidence of Alzheimer's disease.

Other beneficial effects of HRT

- Studies have consistently shown a 20% reduction in the incidence of bowel cancer in women who take HRT compared with those who don't.
- Women using HRT have a lower incidence of stomach cancer.
- Cataracts have been shown to be reduced by 60–80% in women taking HRT.
- Glaucoma (high pressure in the eye) may be less common in women taking HRT.
- Oestrogens seem to protect teeth, possibly by preserving the jaw bone.

The risks of HRT

Blood clots

DVT (blood clots in the leg) is the most significant risk associated with HRT. Pieces of a clot may break off and lodge in a blood vessel in the lungs. This causes a blockage called a pulmonary embolism (PE). Symptoms can include shortness of breath, chest pain when breathing in and coughing up blood.

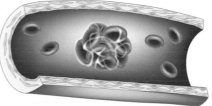

- About 1% of PEs are fatal. Together, DVT and PE are referred to as venous thromboembolism (VTE).
- The risk of VTE is very low in women under 60.
- The risk increases with age. The risk is also increased by lifestyle factors such as obesity and smoking, and being immobile for a long time (for example, on long flights).
- In a study of 1000 women who took oestrogen-only HRT for 5 years during their 50s, 2 had DVT.
- This number increases to 5 per 1000 with combined HRT. However, there is no increased risk if oestrogen is taken as a patch, gel or spray.
- There is also no increased risk of DVT with tibolone, which is sometimes used instead of HRT.

Cardiovascular disease

HRT is known to protect against CVD when started early (see page 33) but women who start HRT after 60 have an increased risk of CVD. This is thought to happen because oestrogen dilates (stretches) the blood vessels, causing the fatty lining in the arteries to break off, which may cause a blockage.

If women do start HRT later in life, the lowest possible dose should be used and, ideally, patches, gel or spray rather than tablets.

Stroke is rare in women under 60 but it is the second most common cause of death in older women. The risk may be reduced by using the lowest dose of HRT, ideally applying it with patches, gel or spray rather than taking tablets.

Gallbladder disease

HRT has been found to increase the risk of gallbladder disease (gallstones and/or gallbladder inflammation). This risk may continue for some years after HRT is stopped. Using oestrogen via the skin as a patch, gel or spray reduces this risk and is therefore recommended for women who are potentially at risk (for example, if you are overweight).

HRT and breast cancer

Many women are concerned about the risk of being diagnosed with breast cancer if they use HRT because research studies have reported conflicting findings, namely that HRT increases, decreases or has no effect on breast cancer risk. This can be very confusing. A major reason for different study results is the different scientific methods used, which can sometimes overly influence positive or negative findings.

Bearing this in mind, current UK advice is as follows.

- Taking oestrogen-only HRT is very unlikely to increase your risk of breast cancer and may even reduce the risk slightly. This is given to women who have had a hysterectomy.

- The risk increases if you are taking combined HRT (oestrogen plus progestogen) but this increased risk only appears to occur in women who have been using combined HRT for a long time (more than 3–4 years). Also, the risk may be less with combined HRT preparations that contain micronised progesterone or dydrogesterone.

- Most women will not be diagnosed with breast cancer if they have previously used HRT (oestrogen-only or combined).

- For women at a low risk of breast cancer (that is, most of the female population), the benefits of using oestrogen-only or combined HRT will exceed potential harms.

- It is useful to think about risk in a balanced fashion. Your risk of being diagnosed with breast cancer is affected by many different things. It may help to know how being overweight and drinking alcohol affect breast cancer risk so that you can see how HRT compares. The table below shows how many additional women would be diagnosed with breast cancer over the next 5 years in a group of 1000 women aged 50–59 when different risk factors are taken into account. The important thing to note is that the excess risk is small, regardless of the risk factor.

Risk of being diagnosed with breast cancer in 1000 women aged 50–59 over the next 5 years

Breast cancer will be diagnosed in 13 women who do not use HRT

- Being overweight: **+4 women**
- Being obese: **+10 women**
- Drinking 4–6 units of alcohol daily: **+8 women**
- Drinking 6 or more units of alcohol daily: **+11 women**
- Taking oestrogen-only HRT for 5 years:

  –6 women (WHI study 2020)
  +3 women (CGHFBC study 2019)
  +3 women (NICE Menopause Guideline 2015)

- Taking combined HRT for 5 years:

  +8 women (WHI study 2020)
  +10 women (CGHFBC study 2019)
  +9 women (NICE Menopause Guideline 2015)

Overweight is defined as a body mass index (BMI) over 25 but less than 30. Obesity is defined as a BMI of 30 or higher.

CGHFBC, Collaborative Group on Hormonal Factors in Breast Cancer; NICE, National Institute for Health and Care Excellence; WHI, Women's Health Initiative. The results from these studies differ because of different methods of data collection.

The data in this table are from Marsden and Pedder (2020) – see 'Find out more' on page 39.

- In women who develop an early menopause, that is, before the age of 50, years of HRT exposure are counted from the age of 50.
- Using certain types of HRT can reduce the risk of bowel cancer, fractures due to osteoporosis (weakened bones) and heart disease (see pages 32–4).
- Regardless of whether a woman uses oestrogen-only or combined HRT, deaths due to all causes are reduced compared with women who have never used HRT.

Some women are concerned about using HRT because of a family history of breast cancer or a previously diagnosed benign breast condition.

- If you have a family history of breast cancer but have not had breast cancer yourself, talk to your GP. They will ask about your family history and may refer you to a specialist family history clinic or a regional genetics centre (depending on where you live). If you are considered to be at low risk after you have been assessed, you can take HRT.
- The only benign breast conditions associated with a significantly increased risk of a breast cancer diagnosis are epithelial atypia and lobular carcinoma in situ. These two conditions can only be diagnosed if a breast biopsy is performed. HRT should be avoided if you have either of these diagnoses, but HRT is probably without risk for all other benign breast conditions.

Key breast cancer facts
- A woman's lifetime risk of being diagnosed with breast cancer is 1 in 8. This sounds worrying but it also means that *most* women (7 in 8) will *never* be diagnosed with breast cancer in their lifetime.
- The main risk factors for being diagnosed with breast cancer (for most women) are being female and older age. Most breast cancers (~80%) are diagnosed in women over 50 years old.
- Postmenopausal lifestyle factors, such as obesity, high alcohol intake and HRT use, are associated with a small increased risk of breast cancer diagnosis. Most women will not be diagnosed as a result of being overweight, drinking alcohol or using HRT.

- Survival rates for breast cancer have improved significantly over the last 50 years, with better treatments and the introduction of the NHS Breast Screening Programme.

- Contrary to popular belief, breast cancer is *not* the major cause of death in postmenopausal women. The greatest cause of death is Alzheimer's disease and dementia, followed by heart disease, stroke, chronic lung conditions and influenza or pneumonia.

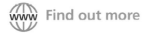 **Find out more**

Marsden J, Pedder H. The risks and benefits of hormone replacement therapy before and after a breast cancer diagnosis. *Post Reprod Health* 2020;26:126–35. Erratum in: *Post Reprod Health* 2021;27:56.

Family history, genes and breast cancer
www.breastcancernow.org/sites/default/files/publications/pdf/bcc32_breast_cancer_in_families_web_pdf.pdf

Breast cancer risk factors
www.womens-health-concern.org/help-and-advice/factsheets/breast-cancer-risk-factors

Leading causes of death, UK: 2001–2018
www.ons.gov.uk/peoplepopulationandcommunity/healthandsocialcare/causesofdeath/articles/leadingcausesofdeathuk/2001to2018

Weighing up the benefits and risks

Use this box to note things you want to discuss with your doctor when deciding about HRT...

Frequently asked questions about HRT

Q: I'm not having many menopausal symptoms, so do I need HRT?

HRT is recommended for most women, because it:
• protects against the development of possible peri-menopausal symptoms in the future
• provides important long-term protection against osteoporosis
• protects the vaginal tissues and bladder.

For women aged up to 60 who are in good health, the benefits of HRT far outweigh any risks.

Q: When should I start HRT?

You can start HRT at any time during the menopause transition. It will help with the symptoms and also provide the long-term benefits we have talked about.

HRT can also be started after the actual menopause and will help with any symptoms that continue. It will also protect the bones from osteoporosis.

However, HRT confers no CVD benefit if it is started outside the window of opportunity (within 5–6 years of the start of the menopause transition).

Q: How long should I take HRT for?

There is no specific age at which you should stop HRT – you can discuss this with your doctor, nurse or pharmacist.

Women are encouraged to take HRT until age 60, to get the full benefits in terms of protection against osteoporosis and CVD.

Women with premature ovarian insufficiency (when the ovaries stop working and no longer produce oestrogen) should continue HRT until at least age 52 (the average age of the menopause).

Q: I couldn't have the contraceptive pill. Can I have HRT?

The levels of hormones in HRT are much lower than in the contraceptive pill. Women who couldn't take the pill (because they have other health conditions or risk factors or side effects) can still take HRT.

Blood pressure increases with age. Oestrogen can raise blood pressure further in some women, but for most women blood pressure remains normal for their age.

Q: What if my symptoms do not improve?

Your doctor will start you on a low dose of HRT, aiming to relieve symptoms with the lowest dose that works for you. You may need to try a higher dose or a different type. Women in their 40s may need higher doses than older women.

Q: What are the side effects of HRT?

The main possible serious side effect of HRT is DVT but the risk is low in otherwise healthy women (see page 35).

Some women experience nausea, breast tenderness and headache when they start taking HRT but this usually passes with time.

Q: Will I put on weight?

HRT does not directly cause women to put on weight. However, hormones can increase appetite, and oestrogen can cause fluid retention, which will increase bodyweight.

You need fewer calories as you get older, because your metabolism slows down, so it is important to reduce your calorie intake to make sure that you don't put on weight.

Tips for partners

Partners can find the menopause a challenging time too – even though they want to support you, they may not know how to. Encourage them to read the following tips and check out the suggested websites for more information.

- Learn about the menopause (this booklet is a good place to start) – the more you know, the more you can support your partner.
- Talk about it – make time to ask your partner how she's feeling and what she's going through.
- Ask – "What can I do to support you?" or "What do you need?"
- Get practical – can you help with some of the things your partner normally does, particularly if she's feeling overwhelmed? Small acts can make a huge difference.
- Take a step back – remember that mood swings and irritability can be part of the menopause, so try to resist snapping back.
- Offer reassurance – many women lose their self-confidence during the menopause; tell your partner that she looks good.
- Don't take it personally – intimate relationships often suffer during the menopause. Just because your partner does not want to have sex does not mean she's rejecting you.
- Be patient – things do get better.

---

www Find out more

There's lots of advice online – these websites are a good place to start:

www.menopausesupport.co.uk/?p=1700

www.femalefirst.co.uk/health/how-to-support-a-partner-through-the-menopause-1214180.html

www.everydayhealth.com/menopause/a-mans-guide-to-menopause.aspx

www.relate.org.uk/relationship-help/help-relationships/feeling-unsatisfied-your-relationship/menopause-affecting-our-relationship-how-do-i-talk-my-partner

---

Menopause and the workplace

You may feel reluctant to discuss the menopause with your employer, but increased openness about the menopause means that more employers understand how it may affect their staff. Often, a few simple changes can help you continue to perform your role successfully.

How do I raise the subject?

If you don't feel comfortable approaching your line manager/employer directly, is there someone else in your workplace that you would be happy to talk to? Some organisations have menopause or wellbeing champions, but you could also talk to a member of the human resources team, a trade union representative or an occupational health specialist if your employer has one.

Whoever you choose to talk to, it's worth scheduling in some time to do so and booking a private room for the conversation if you can. Prepare what you want to say, rehearse it mentally (or with a friend if you prefer) and think about the changes that could make your life more comfortable.

What adjustments might my employer consider?

- Working hours: if you are struggling with lack of sleep, is it possible to change your working hours or adjust your shift patterns or work from home?
- Breaks: can you be allowed to take breaks when you need them, or regular breaks in a more private space where you can manage your symptoms?
- Ventilation: could you have a desk fan, sit nearer a window that opens or adjust the air conditioning?
- Toilets: if you need easy access to the toilets, could you move your desk nearer to them?

- Clothing/uniform: is there any flexibility on company requirements so that you can choose what you wear? For instance, do you have to wear a jacket at all times? Can you avoid uniforms made of synthetic fibres, or wear a looser uniform that is more comfortable?

Because the symptoms of the menopause will fluctuate, it's worth reviewing any adjustments regularly with your employer and discussing and agreeing other changes if you need them.

Find out more

Advice on discussing the menopause with your employer:

www.henpicked.net/menopause-how-to-have-confident-conversations-with-your-manager/

General advice for employers and employees:

www.acas.org.uk/guidance-for-employers-to-help-manage-the-impact-of-menopause-at-work

www.fom.ac.uk/wp-content/uploads/Guidance-on-menopause-and-the-workplace-v6.pdf

---

My notes

Make a note here of issues you would like to raise with your employer...

Breaking the taboo and getting support

The menopause transition is a significant milestone, marking the end of the reproductive years. For some women this may be tinged with sadness, whereas others may embrace a newfound freedom from periods and the worry of pregnancy.

Although the menopause transition can have a marked effect on women's working, home and social lives, the menopause is a natural process and it does not have to be unpleasant.

Fortunately, awareness of perimenopausal symptoms and the challenges that some women face during the menopause transition is improving all the time. It is receiving media attention, helped by celebrities talking about their own experiences.

The International Menopause Society (IMS) launched World Menopause day in 2014 to raise awareness of the issues and it has been held yearly since, each time focusing on a different issue.

Talking helps!

It is important to talk to people. The more open we are, the easier it becomes.

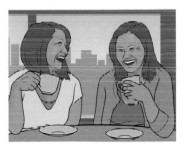

Talk to your partner and children about how you feel; they can be more supportive if they know what you are going through.

If sex is uncomfortable or painful, tell your partner. Comfort and affection are important, even if you don't feel like having sex.

Your peer group may also be hiding symptoms. Talking or laughing about experiences of hot flushes for example, may help you all feel better!

What's new?

- HRT products containing Estetrol (E4) are being evaluated in trials. Estetrol acts like oestrogen on the vagina, womb, bone and brain but blocks the effects of oestrogen in breast tissue. Estetrol may have less effect on the risk of developing blood clots.
- Medications called neurokinin 1/3 receptor antagonists are being developed for the treatment of hot flushes.
- The British Menopause Society has developed a training course on cognitive behavioural therapy (CBT) for doctors, nurses and other healthcare professionals to help them give better support to women who experience problematic symptoms during the menopause transition.
- Menopause cafés are being set up across the UK – forums for women to discuss their experiences (www.menopausecafe.net).
- Laser treatment for urogenital atrophy is available in the private sector and may be offered as an NHS treatment in future.
- Menopause workshops are being run by various organisations – it is wise to check the qualifications and credentials of people running such workshops.

Useful resources

Menopause Matters: menopausematters.co.uk
(magazine and website, including advice for the men in your life!)

British Menopause Society: thebms.org.uk

International Menopause Society: www.imsociety.org

NHS: www.nhs.uk/conditions/menopause

Women's Health Concern: www.womens-health-concern.org
(the patient arm of the British Menopause Society)

Glossary

BMS: British Menopause Society

CVD (cardiovascular disease): heart attack and stroke

DHEA (dehydroepiandrosterone): a hormone that converts in the body into oestrogen.

DVT (deep vein thrombosis): blood clot in the veins of the leg

Early menopause: menstrual periods stop before the age of 45

FSH (follicle-stimulating hormone): a key hormone in the menstrual cycle that triggers the maturation (ripening) of an ovum (egg)

HRT (hormone replacement therapy): medication, also known as menopausal hormone treatment (MHT), containing oestrogen, either alone or with a progestogen; it is used to relieve symptoms during the menopause transition and protect against the long-term effects of the menopause

Hysterectomy: surgical removal of the uterus (womb)

IUS (intrauterine system): a device inserted into the neck of the womb to provide contraception and control heavy bleeding; the Mirena IUS releases low levels of a progestogen and can be used in HRT

Libido: sex drive or desire for sexual activity

Menopause: specifically, the last menstrual period

Menopause transition: the gradual change as oestrogen levels decrease and periods stop (also known as peri-menopause)

Oestrogen: a key hormone released by the ovaries; loss of oestrogen as the ovaries age causes the menopause

Osteoporosis: thinning of the bone (which can occur when oestrogen levels are low after the menopause)

Perimenopause: the years around the menopause when oestrogen levels are decreasing

Postmenopause: starts 12 months after the menopause (last menstrual period)

Premature ovarian insufficiency (POI): failure of the ovaries before age 40

Progesterone: a natural hormone that helps regulate the menstrual cycle

Progestogen: medication that is similar to natural progesterone, used in HRT

Sequential HRT: hormone replacement therapy that contains a progestogen for 12–14 days of each 28-day cycle, allowing a monthly withdrawal bleed

Tibolone: a medication that has similar effects to oestrogen and progesterone that may be used to relieve symptoms during the menopause transition

Vaginal dryness: loss of oestrogen causes the tissues of the vagina to become dry and less stretchy, so they are more easily damaged

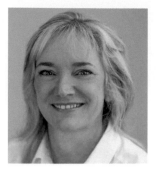

By **Paula Briggs**
MBchB FRCGP FFSRH Gynae Dip Venereology
Consultant in Sexual and Reproductive Health,
Liverpool Women's NHS Foundation Trust; and
Medical Advisory Council, The British Menopause Society.

Although this booklet has been supported by
pharmaceutical funding, the opinions expressed are
those of the Editor.

Theramex has provided funding for this educational material. Theramex has had no
editorial input into the content of this material.

With thanks to **Jo Marsden**, Medical Advisory Council, The British Menopause Society,
and **Hugo Pedder**, Population Health Sciences, University of Bristol, for their additional
content on HRT and breast cancer risk.

© 2021 in this edition, S. Karger Publishers Limited
ISBN: 978-3-318-07001-9

Questions for the Editor

How has this book helped you? Is there anything you didn't understand?
Do you still have any unanswered questions? Please send your questions,
or any other comments, to fastfacts@karger.com
and help readers of future editions. Thank you!

With sincere thanks to those who have reviewed this publication
for all their help and guidance
